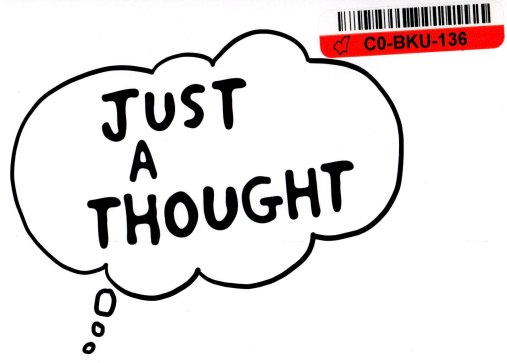

Uncensored Narratives on Teen Mental Health

RESEARCHED AND EDITED BY
THE CHC TEEN WELLNESS COMMITTEE
MENTORED BY KATHERINE REEVES, PMHNP-BC AND CHRISTINE WANG, MA

PUBLISHED BY CHC | PALO ALTO, CA

Just a Thought: Uncensored Narratives on Teen Mental Health
Published in 2018 by
Children's Health Council
650 Clark Way
Palo Alto, CA 94304 USA
www.chconline.org

CHC Teen Wellness Committee mentored by Katherine Reeves, PMHNP-BC and Christine Wang, MA
Book researched, designed and edited by CHC Teen Wellness Committee
Cover design and typesetting by Keira Dooley, Design by Dooley
Copy editing by Angie Mansfield
Illustrations used with permission of Gemma Correll

Paperback ISBN: ISBN 978-0-692-12772-8

Printed in the United States of America
Second Printing: 2018
CHC | Palo Alto, California

DEDICATION

This book is dedicated to all of those who have been affected by mental illness, to those who have inspired us to improve the mental health of teens and to those whose voices have not yet been heard.

—The CHC Teen Wellness Committee

ACKNOWLEDGEMENTS

We want to thank all the courageous teens that poured their honesty into our surveys. Their candid voices brought this book to life, and they are the reason that this work matters.

We would also like to thank the Teen Wellness Committee's advisors, Katherine Reeves and Christine Wang. From organizing bi-weekly meetings to garnering funding for the book, we sincerely appreciate their unconditional support throughout this project.

Gemma Correll's illustrations added a very special touch to this book, and we cannot thank her enough for her amazing artwork.

The CHC Teen Wellness Committee

Maya Chawla
Ethan Du
Nadia Ghaffari
Niklas Goodman
Kiley Haberkorn
Caden Hansen
Danny Howell
Hamsa Jambulapati
Hei Man (Hazel) Lam
Theresa Lim

Madeline Lurie
Ananya Iyer
Meghna Raman
Renée Remsberg
Lindsay Royse
Meghna Singh
Emily Snelling
Kaia Stannard-Stockton
Hannalei Wilson

The CHC Book Advisory Team

Katherine Reeves, PMHNP-BC
Christine Wang, EdM

Special thanks to Dr. Ramsey Khasho, Chief Clinical Officer at CHC and Liza Bennigson, Content Marketing Manager.

THANK YOU

This book could not have been completed without the relentless emotional and financial support of countless concerned community members who advocate for teens on a daily basis. We offer our heartfelt thanks and appreciation to these heroes and hope this book will shed further light on the issues of teen mental health and wellness and offer a way forward.

TABLE OF CONTENTS

TRIGGER WARNING: This book discusses difficult mental health issues. Be aware that the comments in this book, though authentic, are raw and uncensored. They may shock or surprise. We hope they will prompt frank and honest discussions between parents, teens, friends and educators about important topics relating to teen mental health. If you are currently in crisis, Text HELLO to 741741. Additional mental health and crisis resources are available on page 86.

Nineteen teenagers from 12 high schools in the San Francisco Bay Area met in September 2017 at Children's Health Council (CHC) in Palo Alto, California to talk about mental health.

Over the course of nine months, they created this book, *Just a Thought*, to express their opinions about the mental health struggles teens face in high school. This is a collection of quotes taken directly from teen survey responses and narration by high school students commenting on the reports of their peers.

We are confronted daily with reasons teens may hide their experiences with mental illness. The comments in this book break that barrier. They are raw, unfiltered, and allow the reader to appreciate both the strengths and gaping holes in the health and education systems responsible for taking care of these kids. **Teens tell us in this book, in their own words, how we might help.**

The group of teenagers who put this book together came to CHC, a community nonprofit that provides mental health and education services, with the mutual goal to advocate for kids suffering with mental illness. They became the Teen Wellness Committee at CHC. They met bi-weekly to voice ideas, develop solutions, and take action to address mental health concerns.

Each of the 19 teens was unique. We had freshmen navigating high school social situations for the first time, a founder of a mental health start-up, several seniors applying to college, an athlete worried about being sweaty in meetings and kids with parents who wondered whether something related to computer science might be a more practical extracurricular. Some of the teens had struggled themselves with mental illness, many had watched friends navigate mental health treatment, and a few had even lost loved ones to suicide. But all of them knew the difficulties teens face when dealing with mental health issues. And all of them thought teens needed to be heard.

This book contains the voices of teens – entirely in their own words. The group developed a forty-question survey that was sent out via Instagram, Facebook and Snapchat. They received hundreds of survey responses that contained thousands of comments. The teens reviewed and distilled the comments into four major themes – things teens would like to say to friends, teachers, parents and themselves.

The mental health of teens is a growing concern. According to the National Alliance on Mental Illness (NAMI), approximately 1 in 5 youth aged 13–18 (21.4%) experiences a severe mental disorder at some point during their lifetime.[1]

[1] "Mental Health By The Numbers." National Alliance on Mental Illness (NAMI), July 2018.
https://www.nami.org/learn-more/mental-health-by-the-numbers.

According to the Centers for Disease Control, suicide is the second leading cause of death in youth between 10 and 24 years old, resulting in the death of about 6,000 young people each year. [2] Along with those who completed suicide, 16% of teens who responded to a nationwide survey reported seriously considering suicide in the twelve preceding months.[3] And in the last decade, the mental health of kids in the US has continued to worsen. Between 2007 and 2017, the suicide rate of girls between 15 and 19 years old doubled; it increased by 13% in boys of the same age.[4]

The teens that compiled this book were acutely aware of the increasing prevalence of suicide. CHC's home town of Palo Alto, CA has experienced two suicide clusters in the past decade. Those losses have left our community reeling. Our teens are leading the effort to focus on changing the trajectory for those youth still struggling with a mental disorder before things get worse.

Experts continue to publish important reports highlighting new mental health data and the science behind illnesses, but there are few accounts of teens' experiences in their own words. These teens agreed to share their experiences, as well as those of their peers, in hopes of breaking down misconceptions and increasing community understanding of teen mental health. We are exceedingly proud of the grit, passion and honesty the group showed with this project and are brought to tears by the hope they exude as they discuss what's next for the future of teen mental health.

Katherine Reeves, PMHNP-BC
Psychiatric Mental Health Nurse Practitioner
Children's Health Council, Palo Alto, CA

[2] "Suicide: Suicide is a leading cause of death in the United States." The National Institute of Mental Health Information Resource Center, National Institute of Mental Health, May 2018, https://www.nimh.nih.gov/health/statistics/suicide.shtml.

[3] "Gateway to Health Communication & Social Marketing Practice." Centers for Disease Control and Prevention, 15 Sept. 2017, www.cdc.gov/healthcommunication/toolstemplates/entertainmented/tips/SuicideYouth.html.

[4] "Morbidity and Mortality Weekly Report (MMWR)." Centers for Disease Control and Prevention, 3 Aug. 2017, www.cdc.gov/mmwr/volumes/66/wr/mm6630a6.htm.

TO FRIENDS

REACHING OUT AND SEEKING HELP

How do you know if it's okay to reach out?

One of the most difficult parts of being a friend to someone struggling is knowing when to reach out for help. Mental health can be a roller coaster and, as a result, can affect the people who are helping the most.

We asked many of our fellow teens when they thought they should seek help for friends, and the most common answer was this:

"If your friend is showing signs of depression, is self-harming, or has suicidal thoughts."

Others said that they could tell it was time to reach out when their friend was not "acting like their usual self." For some people, that's obvious. For others, it can be harder to tell.

Another take on this question approached the "you" aspect, and how to use your own feelings to figure it out.

"When helping them with their issues starts to hinder your own mental health."

Sometimes it may be unclear whether or not it's appropriate to reach out. When a life may be on the line, you should play it safe.

Reaching out is a really, really hard thing to do. But it's always better to lose a friendship than to lose a friend. And a good rule of thumb:

"If you're even wondering whether it's time to reach out, then yes, it's time."

SELF CARE REWARD STICKERS

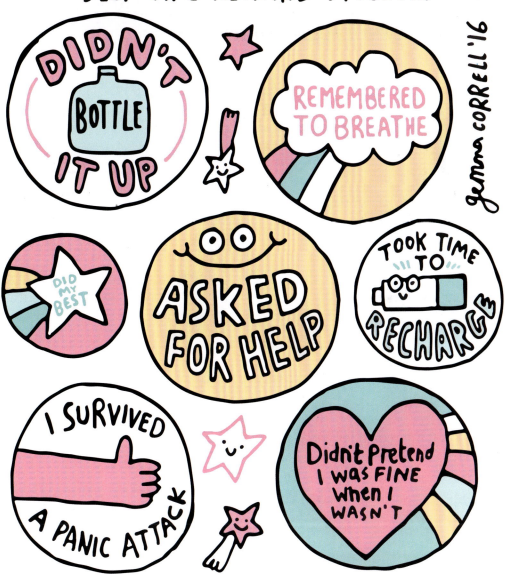

1

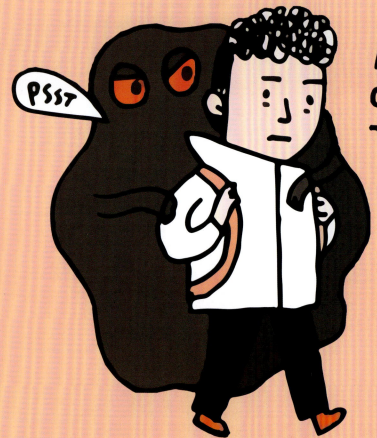

WHEN SHOULD A FRIEND REACH OUT
Teens explain what they think is appropriate and share their stories

When should a friend reach out? When should they tell an adult? Is it okay to tell adults something your friend has confided in you?

These questions all boil down to the same thing: is it okay to share information that a friend has asked you not to share?

"Their honesty is what saved them."

The bottom line is this: if a friend is thinking about hurting themselves, you need to seek outside support. Find a trusted adult, or visit the resource list on page 86 of this book. For other concerns, determine boundaries and expectations with your friends now. The impact may be greater than you imagine.

STORY SHARING
Teens' specific experiences with friends

"One day I was feeling particularly suicidal and talked to my friend about it. She called my mom immediately and told her my location. It was helpful. I'm alive and happy. In the moment I was angry and I felt betrayed, but...you would rather want the person alive and angry at you than dead."

Have you ever considered suicide?

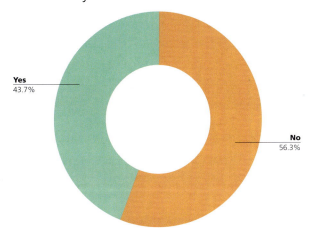

Yes
43.7%

No
56.3%

LETTER FROM A TEEN TO A PEER

To the girl who saw me,

I know. I know I'm lying on the ground. I know that my entire body is shaking as if I were an earthquake. I know you can hear me gasping for air like I'm trapped underwater. You don't think I can see you staring as a school administrator attempts to move me from the floor of the hallway to the counselor's office. I can see it in your eyes: you think I'm just being dramatic. That the reason I keep collapsing onto the ground is for attention. I know you don't understand what is going on or why, so here I am, hoping to give you a solid explanation.

I am having a panic attack, which is exactly what it sounds like. My brain has become so overcome with anxiety that my body physically cannot handle it.

They're different for everyone. Some people remain frozen, paralyzed by the panic. Others dissociate completely, hoping that by removing themselves from reality all the worry will go away. And others have different reactions still. I, however, explode. **I start to hyperventilate, because it feels the air has been knocked out of me, and I can't breathe.** I begin to cry, because I'm so overwhelmed I don't know what else to do. I collapse on the ground, because my legs are so numb and I can't hold myself up.

With my anxiety disorder, it's as if my mind is caught in a whirlpool of worry. Sometimes I can keep it under control and I feel normal, almost content. But other times, I can't help getting sucked in. My thoughts begin to spiral and I feel as if I am falling in. Sometimes no matter how hard I try, no matter how hard I fight off a panic attack, I can't control it.

Trying to prevent a panic attack is one of the most difficult things I've had to do. There is so much running through my head, each thought trying to take control over the last. **There's all this energy in my body, and I'm struggling to control it all.** It's exhausting. It's so, so exhausting.

I used to have attacks 3-4 times a week, often during school. I would get overwhelmed and run out of my classes, collapsing onto the ground outside. **I would endure many stares like yours. People looking at me as if I was broken, as if I should've been able to control myself.** Teachers confused and unsure what they were supposed to do. School administration frustratingly trying to whisk me off to the office, telling me that I was a disturbance to class and needed to get my stress under control. I was told that I needed to take fewer classes and stop spreading myself so thin. I felt like I was being blamed for my mental illness, as if it was my fault for not being able to function like my peers around me. As if I was just overworking myself, as if it was all in my head.

Panic attacks are not the only part of my anxiety disorder. Anxiety isn't something that just happens a couple times a month, it's something you live with. I constantly pick up nervous habits, like biting my nails or picking at my skin. **I overthink things**, like the stain on my shirt, or the mismatched ceiling tiles, things that most people never think of more than once. I play interactions over and over and over again in my head after they've happened, over-analyzing body language and intonation.

Even before the attacks, my friends noticed that something was wrong, and after the panic attacks began, they became even more worried. They tried to help me, and I pushed them away. **I thought I could handle it by myself, and that by asking for help I was giving up**. I thought asking for help made me weak. But after the third attack, I decided I needed to get help, real help. I went to my general physician, who sent me to a psychiatrist that put me on selective serotonin reuptake inhibitors (SSRIs), hoping that these anti-anxiety meds would stop the attacks. After two months on the medication, I realized that the medication was doing me more harm than good. Although the attacks stopped, my depression became increasingly worse. During these months, I was also seeing a therapist. After I stopped taking the medication, **she helped with both my anxiety and depression disorders by teaching me to be mindful and use coping mechanisms.** She finally diagnosed me with Generalized Anxiety Disorder and Major Depressive Disorder. Putting a name to my problems felt validating, because it made me realize that it wasn't all in my head.

It's been a year since all this happened, since you saw me in the hallway, and I'm happy to report I am feeling better. While I'm still living with my mental illness, I no longer have panic attacks all the time. I know I can be an active member of society, regardless of my mental illness, and I am.

I know you didn't mean any harm when you first saw me, but it's people who haven't experienced mental illness who make people like me, who are struggling, feel stigmatized and alone. I know it's not your fault or mine, but that of the education system. It's the fault of those before us who have stigmatized mental illness, those who have shunned people like me into silence.

I hope my story provides those who read it with a perspective of mental health they haven't heard before. I hope you realize that it's time to end the stigma, so that people like me can come forward with their stories, so that the next generation doesn't have to go through the same thing I had to.

Best,
Your Classmate

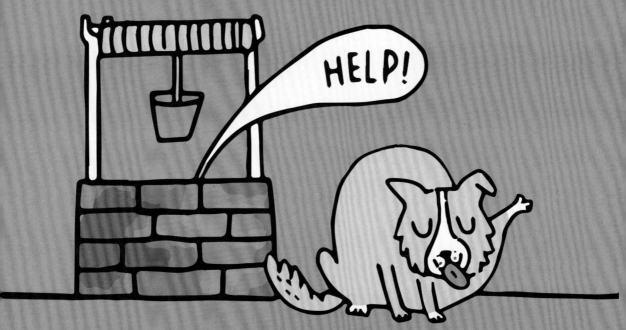

WHAT DISCOURAGES TEENS FROM REACHING OUT?

Teens share what they think about before reaching out for help

Asking for help is always tough. But there are also things that might discourage a teen from reaching out; we asked other teens what they thought those were.

"Judgement. Betraying someone else's trust."

One common fear is that by reaching out, you could be betraying your friend's trust. While it's likely your friend won't be happy about it at first, remember that what you're doing is for their mental health. As a teen, you have limited resources, so no one expects you to solve these problems on your own.

Teens mentioned other factors too.

"Adults want to keep their institution's reputation safe."

It may seem like a school's reporting procedures are not aligned with what you need in the moment. But if you don't reach out, you could be dismissing potential help. By voicing your needs and advocating for yourself, you're helping to make it clear to those adults that these issues are important and should not be disregarded.

So what's the general rule? How do you decide? As one teen put it:

"It's better to lose a friendship than a friend."

In general, keep your friend's best interests in mind and help advocate for them when appropriate. In situations like these, trust yourself and think carefully about the way that you reach out.

SUPPORT FROM FRIENDS

The best and worst ways that teens can help support their friends

Friends are often our go-to support network. They're like us. They understand. They know us. So how can friends help out? The most typical response:

"Just be there for me."

Some people want hugs, others just want to talk. Some people don't want any special treatment—they just want to go about life. One concrete example:

"Ask me what's going on. Invite me to social gatherings."

The truth is, support looks different for every person. So communicate with your friends about what works for you; support from friends can be crucial.

Teens also gave us some examples of what's not supportive.

"Don't invalidate my issues."

When someone's going through a tough time, they often need a friend who will listen. That means listening without interrupting and just giving them one hundred percent attention for a minute or two. Don't say that your friend is being too "complainy" or compare their problems to your own. Just listen to what they have to say.

What's the underlying message? How can you be a supportive friend? What is it we truly want from our friends? It's straightforward:

"I want my friends to encourage me and make me feel like I matter to them."

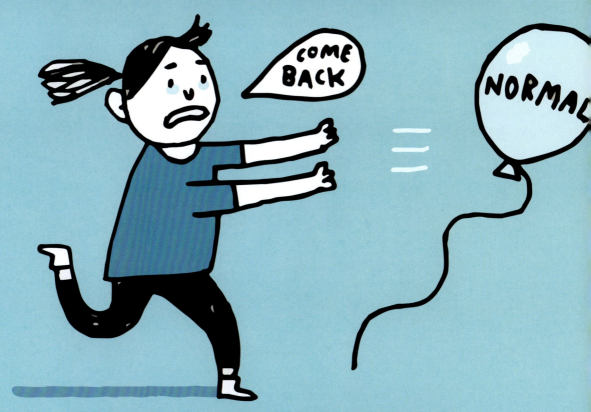

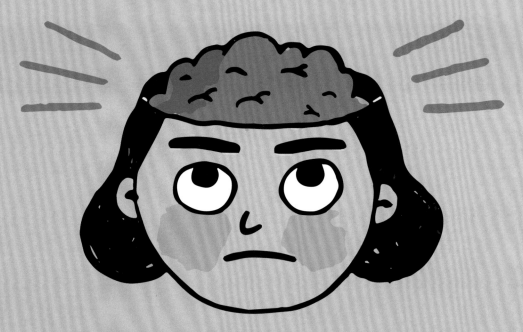

DOS AND DONT'S

In teens' words, what friends should and should not do

DOS

"Just be kind, and know that sometimes I need to be left alone."

"Check in with me every so often... it helps when the other person prompts the conversation."

"Do what's right for me, whether or not that may affect our friendship."

"I don't need a comforter but a problem solver."

DONT'S

"Don't invalidate my issues."

"If you're not close enough to a person for you to really know what's going on, leave it to someone who is."

"Don't pressure me to talk when I'm not wanting to."

"Don't change your actions or treatment of me."

"Don't question my experiences."

"Don't flat out tell me that I sound like I'm complaining too much."

PROMOTING TEEN MENTAL HEALTH
How can friends help?

Teen mental health is a complicated thing that many people often misunderstand. As a society, we are seeking positive change. From campaigns to committees, teens all around the world are working to promote mental health in teens.

To expand on this, we asked teens what they thought friends could do. The responses often said the same thing.

"Be supportive and open."

Whether it be "talking to others about it and being more open" or "checking in and making sure everyone is doing well," teens just want support from their friends.

It's also important to recognize that friends often go to each other when in times of need.

"Help someone who needs help. Don't make a scene."

For teens, confiding in one another takes a lot of trust. It also means that in times of need, our friends sometimes have to make hard decisions or to be the voice of reason in a difficult situation. What does that mean for the friend?

"It's not your job to fix your friend's problem. It's the support that matters."

In other words, take time to listen, be open and know that you can always talk to a trusted adult when the situation feels out of your control.

#MENTALILLNESSFEELSLIKE

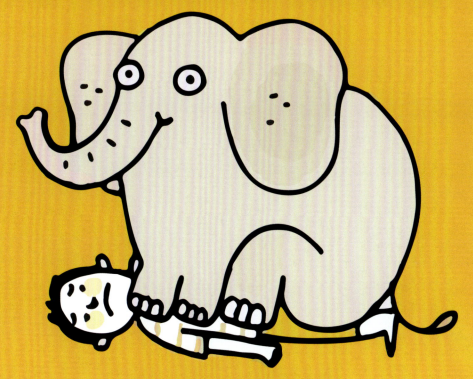

AN ELEPHANT
SITTING ON YOUR CHEST
#ANXIETY

Gemma CORRELL

TO PARENTS

IMPACTFUL RELATIONSHIPS
Teens share the specific impact parents have on their mental health

Parents can be our greatest support system. Most of our fellow teens expressed gratitude towards their parents for their emotional support, and appreciated their patience and listening skills.

"They told me they love me and to look at the positive things in life."

Teens also felt more comfortable when parents allowed them to make their own decisions, rather than embodying the traditional "helicopter parent."

"Just listen to me... without pushing too much or prying."

We often overlook parental support as unimportant, when in reality we teens look to our parents for approval.

"When I was worried in college about failing a class and called them, they told me it's okay if I fail, that they will love me no matter what."

Additionally, teens appreciated their parents' efforts to put them in therapy.

"My parents hooked me up with a dope ass therapist."

Teens most often go to their parents seeking love, support and advice, and all they ask is that their parents are willing to offer those three things.

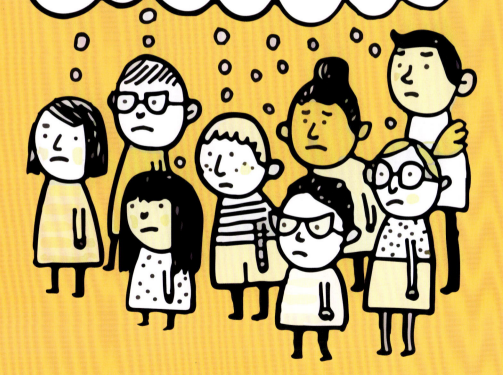

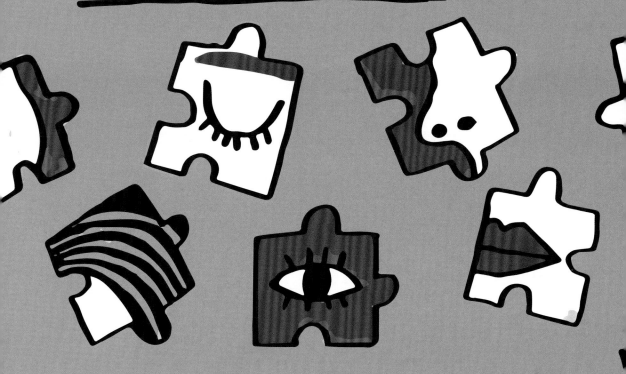

BIPOLAR DISORDER FEELS LIKE...

"KNOWING YOU HAVE ALL THE PIECES
BUT FINDING IT IMPOSSIBLE TO
REMEMBER HOW THEY FIT TOGETHER"

#MENTALILLNESSFEELSLIKE
Gemma CORRELL

PARENTS: HOW THEY CAN HELP

Teens explain the helpful things parents have done for their mental health

"Reassured me that they are okay with what I'm going through and do not judge me for it."

"Been a stable support system and always made me feel like they'll be there and be proud."

"My parents never worried about my grades but instead always reinforced to me that they wanted me to be healthy."

"When my friends were struggling, I was able to confide in my mom. She guided me to make the right decisions and advised me when it was time to tell a professional who could do more."

"Checked in with me."

"Put me in therapy!"

"Always offering to listen without pushing too much or prying."

1

"I became really depressed all throughout 8th grade. I don't know how it started or why, but I felt lethargic a lot more and I was inexplicably sad for things that didn't usually make me sad. Then when things legitimately made me sad, my reaction was a lot stronger than usual, but **my mom would yell at me all the time 'to stop being too negative' or 'stop being in a dark cloud.'** When I had issues with friends like every normal middle schooler, **she would tell me that 'no one liked me because I was so dark all the time' and that 'I would never be able to make friends in high school.'"**

WHAT HELPS AND WHAT DOESN'T

Teens share specific experiences demonstrating both good and bad responses

"I was crying really hard one night and my mother didn't do anything really. She just sort of reinforced my fears about myself. She does this often."

"My parents are different than most, and they always have my back... I always tell my parents how I'm doing. They're my support."

"I used to be larger than a lot of other girls in my grade... I told my mom how I was feeling, and she told me how beautiful I am and that I should never worry about my weight."

"I went to my mother and told her that I had been contemplating suicide. She told me that it was fine, and I didn't have anything to worry about."

"I just told my parents that I had gone to the wellness center because I was feeling depressed. And we had a great conversation about it, which led to me getting help."

"They were angry with me for cutting myself. They don't understand why I feel this way when I have everything in front of me. What they don't understand is that I have the physical support but not emotional support."

WHAT HELPS AND WHAT DOESN'T
Teens share memories of specific moments

HELPFUL THINGS PARENTS HAVE SAID

"Do you need a therapist?"

"Reassured me that my concerns/cause of mental distress were not something that would affect my future and that I needed to concentrate on being happy."

"That they would do anything to help me feel happy again."

"Mental health is just as important as physical health."

"I'm here for you no matter what."

"Said that they were open to talk about anything with me with no judgment."

"Grades won't be written on your gravestone."

"To take a step back and relax."

"Expressing love."

UNHELPFUL THINGS PARENTS HAVE SAID

"I hate when you act like this."

"It's just stress."

"Don't pull an 'anxiety card.'"

"You're just asking for attention."

"That receiving outside help doesn't work,
and mental issues are best solved internally."

"Called me lazy when I was too depressed to get out of bed for hours at a time."

"That everyone goes through this and I will get over it."

"Avoided it and never talked to me about it."

"You don't have time for that."

DOS AND DONT'S

In teens' words, what parents should and should not do

DOS

"Make sure I'm not overwhelmed in school, promote sleep and exercise."

"Get me help, listen to me."

"Ask me how I'm doing."

"Avoid talking over me or interjecting—just let me talk."

"Tell me you're proud of me."

"Give me alone time."

"Talk to me about it."

"Respect me, try to boost my confidence and strength."

"Letting me take time... to rest."

DONT'S

"Tell me to just get over a problem or acting like it's nothing big."

"Yell at me."

"Tell me I'm making up excuses."

"Not believe me."

"Not sympathize with my feelings."

"Tell me that I'm overreacting at times."

"Be helicopter parents that don't give me any space."

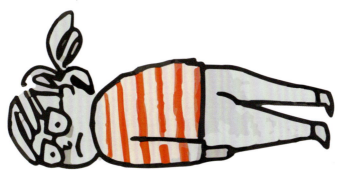

A DEPRESSION

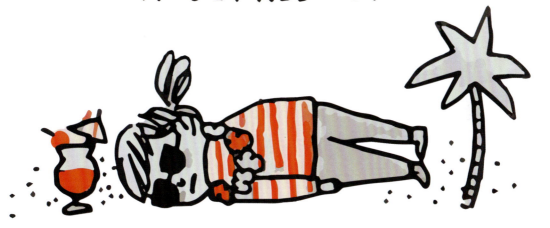

A TROPICAL DEPRESSION

LETTER FROM A TEEN TO HER PARENTS

Dear Mom and Dad,

No words can truly describe my appreciation for everything you have done for me, but this is my best attempt:

I think we all know that, ever since third grade, **I was different from a lot of kids.** I would overthink and worry excessively about everything, especially tests. As soon as you noticed this, you reached out to the counselor at our school to provide me with some help. Looking back now, **I really appreciate that you went out of your way to try to help me**, even though we didn't continue with the counseling. You may not have realized it, but my anxiety continued to develop and get worse as I got older.

Although it was never officially diagnosed, we can all say that we knew I have had this anxiety my entire life. That one day in high school when I had a horrible panic attack was when we realized it was out of control, and something needed to be done about it. Although at first I was frustrated with you for not having gotten me help sooner, it is better late than never. **There is no way I would be as outgoing and comfortable as I am today (even though I am not perfect and definitely still struggle occasionally) if you had not been so open and accepting when I asked if I could see a therapist.** As soon as we had the conversation, you were more than willing to help me find the help I needed. We went to the doctor and I went through an 8-week training.

After, we decided I still needed help so we found a therapist. I know I do not tell you what goes on in my sessions, but let me just tell you: a lot. And all of it has been extremely helpful. I do not know if you have noticed a big difference, but I sure have. Again, I may not be perfect, but the fact that **you were so willing to go past the stigma behind mental health disorders**, acknowledge that I had one, and did everything you could to help me with it is all a child could ask for. You encouraging and supporting my work at the Teen Wellness Committee adds to that, as well. Not many parents can say that they are the ones who helped their child's wellness; in fact, many unfortunately do the opposite.

You both have been extremely pro-wellness and ensure that I am as healthy as I can be, both mentally and physically. **You are able to realize that mental health is just as important as physical health**, and I hope more and more parents can start to realize that as well. I love you both so much. Thank you again for everything, especially all of your support.

Sincerely,
Your daughter

PROMOTING TEEN MENTAL HEALTH
What can parents do to promote teen mental health?

What we teens are looking for is unwavering support from our parents, validation, and for our home to be a safe space. Open conversations about real emotions help destroy the unbearable stigma that surrounds mental health issues.

In addition, simply take time to learn about mental health, and realize the importance of it.

"Parents need to get on board with the fact that mental illness exists and some people...need extra help in order to learn how to handle it."

Once you've had this conversation, use that knowledge in connections with parents and community members to educate others, so they too can understand that it is a reality.

Teens also said that what they wanted most was the freedom to figure out what works best for them.

"Offer your kids options. If they need medication, don't stop them because you don't think it's something you would want for yourself. If they need therapy, give it to them."

Overall, teens want their parents to acknowledge and talk about mental health, and to allow them to have a say in their treatment plans.

Would you feel comfortable going to your parent(s) with a mental health concern?

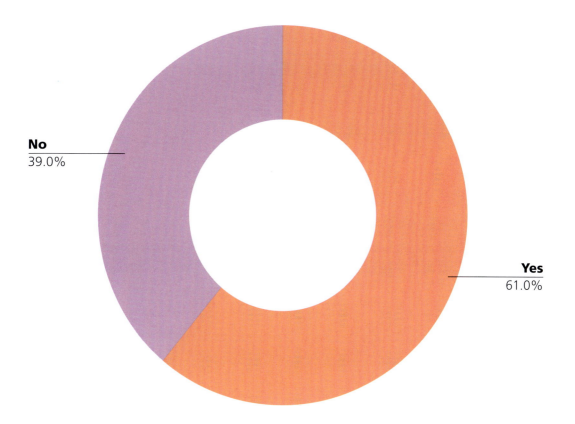

No
39.0%

Yes
61.0%

TO EDUCATORS

Anxie-Trees

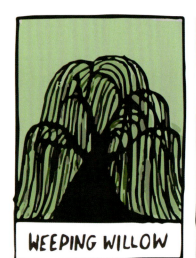

WEEPING WILLOW

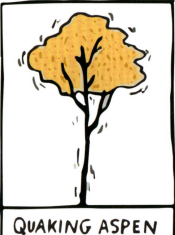

QUAKING ASPEN

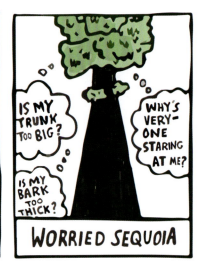

WORRIED SEQUOIA

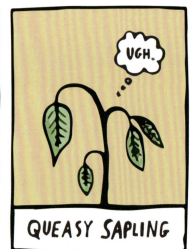

SWEATY PALMS

QUEASY SAPLING

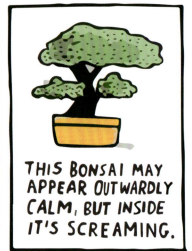

THIS BONSAI MAY APPEAR OUTWARDLY CALM, BUT INSIDE IT'S SCREAMING.

FOUR eyes BY Gemma CORRELL

SCHOOL: TEENS' OPINIONS

Teens share stories of when schools have tried to advocate for mental health

Being one of the most important and prevalent parts of our life, school should be a place where mental health is promoted and where students can talk about it openly. So we asked students how that played out at their schools.

"It never gets talked about but needs to be."

Starting conversations around mental health can be very beneficial, but people often like to pretend that mental health issues aren't affecting their communities. When community members start to discuss mental health, they will be more readily able to get help for the people who need it.

We also asked teens about their experience talking to adults about it.

"When adults don't listen to youth, youth are also unlikely to listen back."

Listening to teens who have personally experienced mental health issues allows educational efforts to accurately portray what it's like to live with these conditions. Also, teens with mental health conditions can feel like they're not being heard. If adults make an obvious effort to listen, teens are more likely to feel respected and valued.

"Schools should listen more closely to students' feedback and should make an effort to incorporate that feedback."

MENTAL HEALTH IN SCHOOL

Teens share the role that school plays in their mental health

School is a huge part of a teen's life. So how does that intersect with mental health? What can schools do to ease the stress that may come with this environment?

"My school is very competitive and makes it difficult not to have anxiety or depression at some point."

Having a competitive or stressful school environment can worsen existing mental health concerns and hinder our ability to maintain mental wellness. Even in the absence of mental health conditions, stress can take a toll.

This being said, there are solutions. We can make many changes (both small logistical ones and larger-scale changes) at the school level to boost students' mental health. Smaller-scale changes can include having late starts and offering students free periods, which allow them to sleep more in the mornings and have more free time.

"Allowing students to leave class for 15 minutes and take a break in our wellness center has been incredible."

Larger changes can have an even greater impact. Letting students have a safe space to deal with mental health issues, or even take a break and rest if they're having a bad day, can be really useful and benefit students' mental health.

#MENTALILLNESSFEELSLIKE

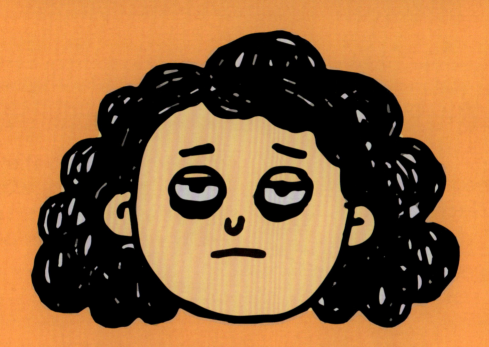

CONSTANT, ACHING
FATIGUE

Gemma CORRELL

SHARE A STORY
Teens discuss how teachers impact mental health

We asked teens to share stories about their interactions with teachers regarding their mental health, and how that conversation may have impacted them as a student or teen.

"They understood perfectly."

There are teachers who are doing everything right, but there are also quite a few who struggle to understand and adequately deal with the mental health challenges that teenagers face.

"Teachers have not had concerns about me and my mental health."

First, teachers need to recognize that mental illness is a reality in their student body and to acknowledge it. For a teenager, knowing that they're being heard is quite powerful. If we know that there is someone open to connecting to us, we'll be more open to reaching out.

"They did not believe that my anxiety was a strong enough excuse and yelled at me for it."

Teachers can sometimes misread the very real, often uncontrollable experiences of youth. When this happens, it can make us doubt if our experiences are valid, and we'll often be less likely to reach out for help. It is important for teachers to be more compassionate and understanding throughout their conversations with us.

"I feel like they didn't want to take the time to help me."

Generally, teachers could build in more accommodation for teens struggling with mental health issues. From reaching out to offer support for a hard project to allowing students to take a moment in the hallway to breathe if they feel anxious, giving students that opportunity can offer relief and reassurance.

"In one of my harder classes, my teacher doesn't think I try... She always calls me out in front of the class and makes me feel even dumber than I am."

Struggling with mental health issues does not mean that we are less intellectual. Teachers sometimes misread uncontrollable symptoms of mental illness as a sign that we are somehow unable to prosper. It is important for teachers to separate someone's mental health from their abilities.

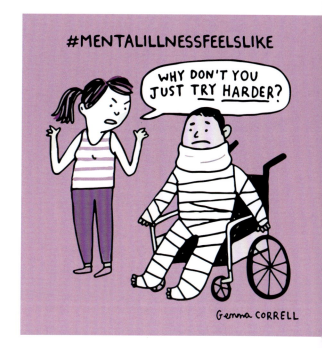

APPROACHING TEACHERS

Teens share what makes teachers approachable regarding mental health

Teachers can be both resources and roadblocks. We asked teens what they thought made teachers approachable, and received a vast range of responses.

"She was calm and had sympathy for me."

Having a trusted teacher who is able to remain calm in difficult times and also listen to students is incredibly important, especially when that teacher may be the only person who the student is sharing their issues with.

"They were open so I was open back."

Opening up is scary, and many teens agreed that by being vulnerable and sharing their own stories, teachers made themselves more approachable and seemed more trustworthy.

"She took time out of her day to check in with me."

It is often the smallest things that can make the largest impact. For students who may not have other resources, knowing that their teacher, someone they may see on a daily basis, is thinking about them and has their best interests in mind can be very comforting.

But not all teens had the same experience:

"Hasn't happened to me."

Overall, students found that they were most able to trust teachers who were open, honest and truly cared.

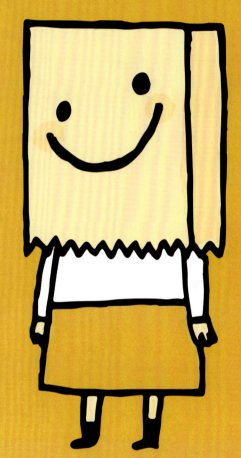

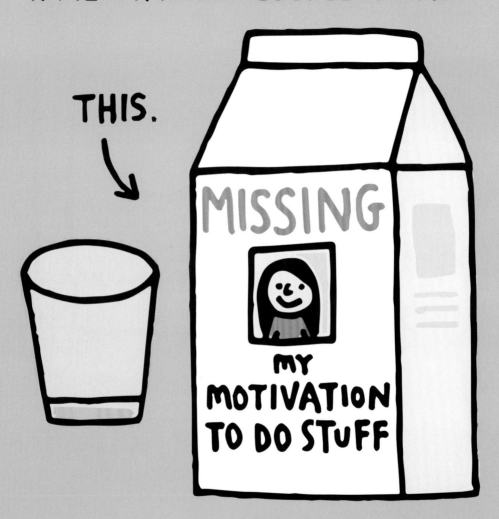

SUPPORT FROM TEACHERS
When and how have teachers supported you and your mental health?

What does it look like when a teacher supports students and their mental health? Teens agreed that being both understanding and available to listen are key.

"I was having a panic attack in class and my teacher found a way to allow me to leave the room."

Some of these are logistical, like allowing students to get an extension on assignments that are stressing them out. However, small acts of kindness can make a big difference.

"My teacher told me to take a break...and write down...all of the things that make me happy."

Also, many students felt that teachers "just listening" was very important. Having a teacher who is willing to sit down and "have a conversation with them and ask how they're feeling" makes students feel "loved and important." Especially for teens who may not have other positive adult role models in their lives, having teachers who believe in them can have a great impact:

"I would not be here today if it wasn't for my teachers."

As adults who interact with students on a day-to-day basis, teachers can greatly affect their students. And it's often the littlest things that create the longest lasting results.

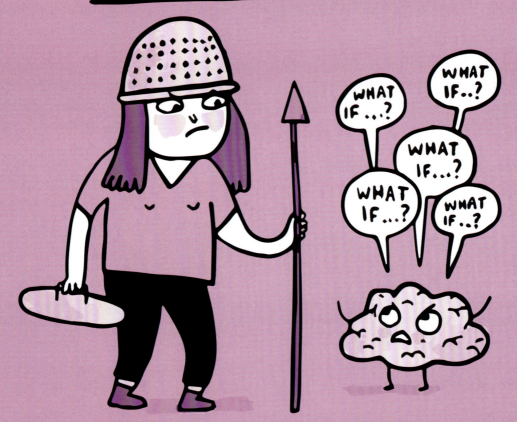

TEENS' MESSAGES TO EDUCATORS

Teens share what they want educators to know about how to support them

"Make your classroom a safe space."

Teens are looking for a trustworthy adult to confide in who will respect their needs and work with them to make classroom accommodations if necessary.

We teens are looking for teachers to be kind and understanding, and to realize how much courage it takes for us to approach an adult and ask for an extension or a break from class. That being said, teens also said this:

"Give students the means to get help."

Reaching out for help is already incredibly difficult. Teachers can help (and also deepen our trust) by offering help when we need or ask for it.

Self-care is especially important. Teens said that by understanding students' needs and advocating for them, educators can play a larger role in teens' mental health.

"Encourage extracurricular activites and allow for that time to be available."

Teens aren't asking for educators to solve mental health issues, but they are asking that educators recognize (and take responsibility for) the impact their actions have on teens. Furthermore, teens just want the time and space to practice self-care and get better. With just a little help, we think that's possible.

DOS AND DONT'S

In teens' words, what educators should and should not do

DOS

"Bring mental health education to middle school, not just high school."

"Encourage extracurricular activities and allow time for that to be available."

"Give students resources and means to get help."

"Give us late passes which cannot be turned into extra credit, which encourages us to use them when we cannot meet a deadline."

DONT'S

"Don't act like something is wrong with me."

"Don't bring unwanted attention to the student! It makes them feel worse!"

"Don't tell me I am too old to be this 'dramatic' about things."

"Stress-free week in school was just a regular stressful week at school but with yoga during lunch. The teachers did not try to lessen the workload at all."

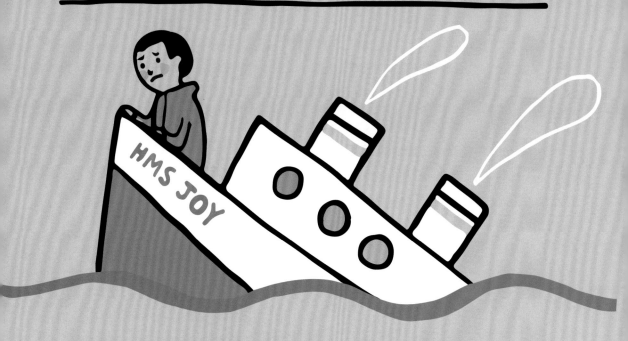

PROMOTING TEEN MENTAL HEALTH

What can teachers do to promote teen mental health?

We asked other teens what they thought educators could do to help promote and advocate for teen mental health.

"Actually listening to the teens completely and fully and trying to understand the whole issue from their point of view."

Listening is more valuable than you might imagine. When we asked other teens, they explained what that meant to them.

"Be more open and easy to talk to—less like a therapist and more like a friend."

Teens also repeatedly mentioned raising awareness. They had requests for when schools should start introducing mental health:

"Bring mental health to middle school, not just high school."

Teens felt that it would be more beneficial to introduce, promote and raise awareness for mental health earlier than high school.

"Raise awareness so that people realize mental illness is a reality and that it is not a bad thing."

PTSD FEELS LIKE ...

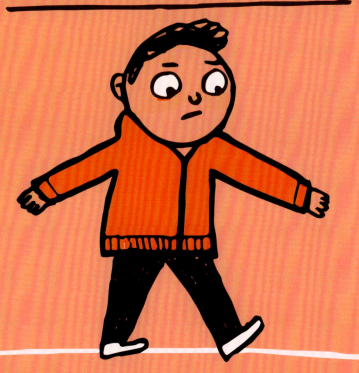

"A NEVER-ENDING TIGHTROPE BETWEEN FIGHT AND FLIGHT"

#MENTALILLNESSFEELSLIKE

Gemma CORRELL

LETTER FROM A TEEN TO A TEACHER

I've had so many good experiences with teachers who've been supportive, but also so many experiences with teachers who, while well-intentioned, haven't actually helped all that much. There are a couple things that have seemed to determine how helpful teachers are.

If I could give advice to my teachers about being supportive of students with mental health conditions, the **first thing I would say is to keep an open mind and stay curious.** We don't expect you to be experts on what we're going through. A lot of other kids like me become self-educated experts on our conditions because we're so used to being misunderstood. Don't fulfill our negative expectations by getting spooked as soon as we say things that you're not familiar with. Ask questions, find resources. I promise that if you say you don't understand something, we'll explain, or if we don't know, we'll be willing to figure it out with you. Be curious and open-minded, and be willing to admit that sometimes you don't know.

Second: trust us. Give us options. Know that we've been made stronger by fighting our demons, and know that when we say something, we mean it. If you empower us by really asking questions and really wanting to hear our opinions, we will be forever grateful. The most stressful situations I've been in have happened because teachers have made decisions without asking me. I know you care. I really, really, know you care. But please at least warn us, okay? Being left out of the loop can feel like salt's being rubbed into an open wound.

Third: know what we actually want. What we want, or at least what I know I want, is to have someone who validates how we feel and shows us that opening up isn't scary. Listen to us, really listen. If we don't ask for advice, assume that we're not asking for advice. Usually all we need is for you to say, "Wow, that sounds hard." At least in my case, if I want advice, I'll ask. Otherwise, just feeling heard is priceless in and of itself.

Fourth: set an example. I know how cliché this is, I really do. It's true, though. Hands down, the most supportive teachers I've had have inspired me to open up through being vulnerable themselves. A big part of why I started to trust people was seeing it modeled through teachers who weren't scared to be vulnerable with their students. That's rare, and I know that. But trust me, it's absolutely priceless.

Be brave, and know that we don't always know what we're doing either. Being a teenager is hard enough, and mental health conditions complicate the whole thing, but having supportive teachers on your side makes it a lot less painful. I know that I have no clue where I'd be without all these amazing people in my life.

—Anonymous

LETTER FROM A TEEN TO A TEACHER

To My Teacher,

Without you, I honestly do not know if I would be able to go to school every day. Knowing you are there every day to have a conversation with is so helpful. It is really hard to find people on campus that I am comfortable talking to, but your classroom has definitely been a safe haven for me. Some things are hard to talk to friends or parents about, so it is really nice to have another advising adult in my life. Opening up is difficult, but I have felt comfortable talking to you about my personal wellness knowing there is no judgment and you will have helpful tips for me. We can talk about anything: school, typical day to day stuff, sports, and most importantly, wellness.

You teach psychology, so that definitely helps, but I really appreciate all the help you have given me with regards to my personal mental health and that of those around me. You have encouraged and helped with a lot of events and other things I have tried to implement on campus. You have supported the work I am doing outside of school by making announcements about it, sharing it with other people, putting posters up in your classroom, helping me organize events, talking to the counseling department, etc. Everything I bring to you is more than just acknowledged; you actually take action!

Many people are afraid to talk to their teachers in general, so the fact that you are so approachable is extremely beneficial. Thank you for everything! I will certainly miss having you around when I am in college, but I will definitely take everything I have learned from you with me.

Sincerely,
Your Student

How many adults on your school campus do you feel comfortable going to with a mental health concern?

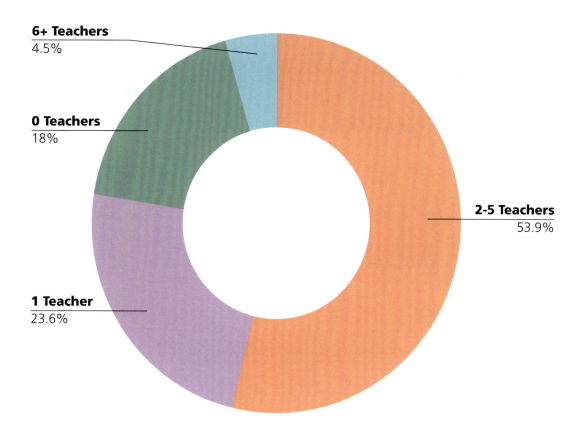

6+ Teachers
4.5%

0 Teachers
18%

2-5 Teachers
53.9%

1 Teacher
23.6%

TO ME

THE REALITY

Teens share some of the real struggles of mental health issues

"I would have anxiety attacks all the time...I never knew that what I was struggling with was anxiety and it took me forever to get help."

"In the past, I've struggled with my self esteem due to being lost about my gender identity and lack of confidence...I find it very difficult to trust myself, open up to others or voice my thoughts to others because of fear of what others think or how I look."

"It is very challenging when you have to deal with PTSD. Everything is a challenge. I find it hard to focus in school and hard to enjoy little things like going out with my friends. It was much worse...when I wasn't getting help and was extremely lonely."

"I was super depressed freshman year, and it killed my grades and a lot of my friendships so I started seeing a therapist and taking medication."

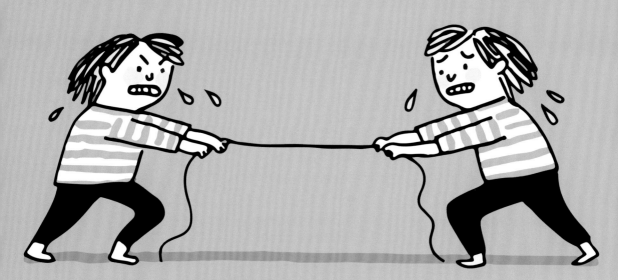

STORIES OF STRESS

Teens share times when stress particularly affected their mental health

Being both a student and an athlete can often make teens feel especially stressed. This massive workload can bury us and degrade our health.

"Baseball meant the world to me and when I had to give it up, I was crushed. But I learned that things happen for a reason...I would have missed out on my youth group and would've been a totally different person."

Many teens described their personal and social interactions with drug use.

"I used to be someone who smoked weed... I began to feel really disengaged in everything that was happening around me and anxious about everything I was doing. I smoked again...thinking I would feel relaxed, yet had a very similar experience, so I stopped smoking completely because it enhanced my anxiety."

Interactions with substance use and even instances of self harm, which are often a call for help, can be taxing to teens on both ends. We have to balance our own needs with the needs of our friends, which can bring additional stress to our lives.

"I had a friend who was cutting and would talk to me about it. Eventually, I went to see a confidential counselor who gave me advice."

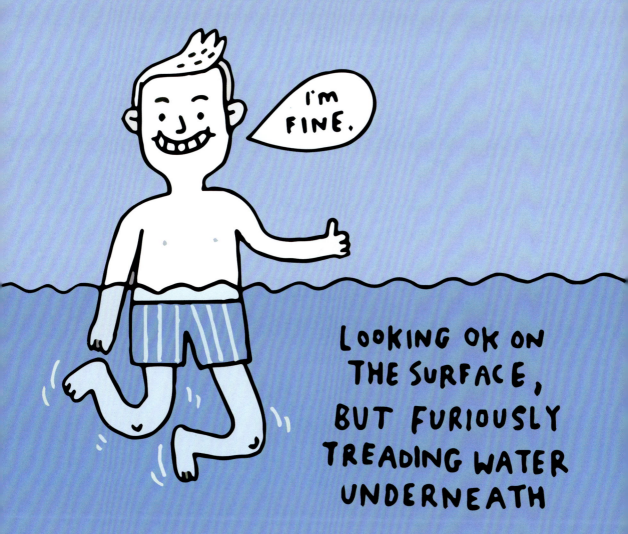

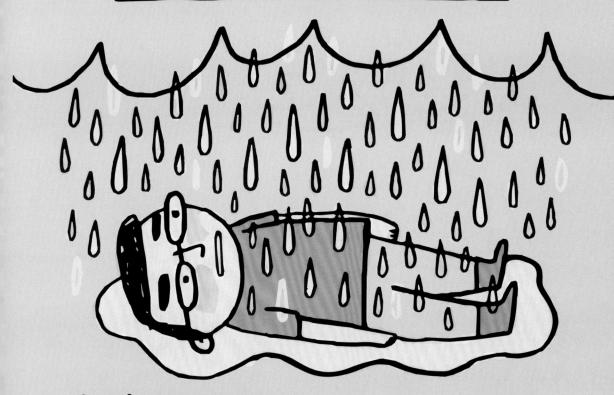

SELF-CARE: FRIENDS AND FAMILY
Teens explain how spending time with others is a form of self-care

We don't always have to practice self-care alone. Often, having the support of our loved ones is powerful. Teens shared the many shapes and forms that that support can take.

"I try to run every day and talk to my friends... as much as I can!"

Along with the company that those close to us can provide, their love is often a reminder of our self worth and can be especially powerful during hardship or difficult times.

"I take care of myself... by reminding myself of how others love me."

Self-care comes with challenges, too; by relying on friends and family, we risk misunderstandings or having our boundaries crossed. A big aspect of self-care is setting those boundaries beforehand so others know when to offer help and when to step back.

"My parents always let me take breaks when I felt I deserved it or needed it, and that's helped me a lot because I know my boundaries and how much I can take before I melt down."

INTERNALLY DRIVEN SELF-CARE
Teens share their internal self-care methods

Self-care is an entirely personal process based each person's individual needs. For this reason, we asked other teens what they did for self-care.

For many teens, gratitude and taking breaks can be integral parts of their self-care routines.

"I take a couple minutes every day to think about things I am grateful for...I let myself spend time watching funny shows and sleeping... and not having to think about anything."

However, it can be hard to be confident in our own worth and it's easy to fall into a self-deprecating mindset. One teen said, "I remind myself that my worth is not defined by my productivity, and that my existence is valuable in and of itself. This often means listening to the voices of my loved ones instead of my inner critics."

"If I'm being honest, I'm still working on that. It's so easy to just stay in bed ...and watch TV. For the longest time I thought that was self care, but it just feeds into the cycle of depression."

It's not always easy. Self-care is something we all have to learn, which often takes time.

"For me, it's doing things like painting my nails, or taking a longer time to do my makeup. Self care... can really help divert the negativity you feel, at least for a little while."

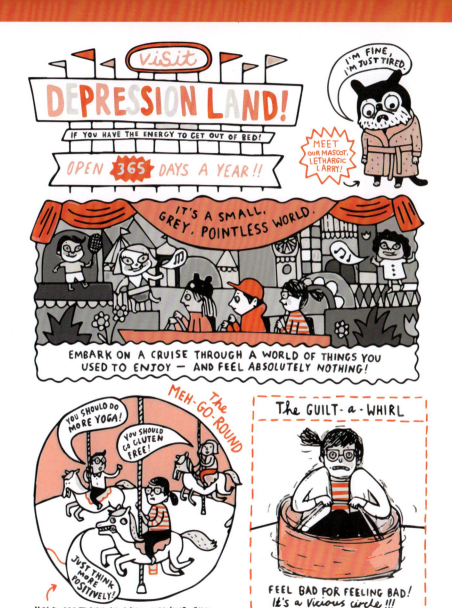

FOUR eyes BY Gemma CORRELL

3

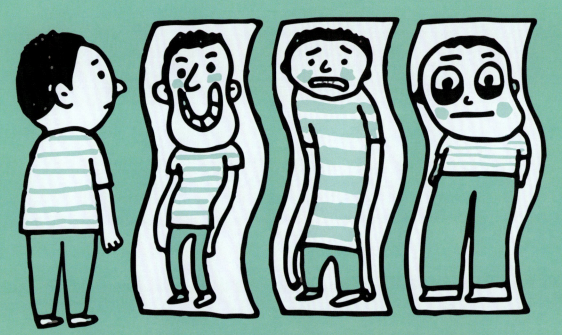

ADVICE TO SELF

Teens share the advice they would give to their younger self

"It will all work out in the end."

"Focus on yourself more than the superficial things."

"Self harm will never make you feel good about yourself."

"Breathe and make sure you keep time for the things you love to do."

"Therapy works."

"Things will definitely get better."

"Ask for help even if you think you can do it by yourself. You are strong and asking for help does not say otherwise."

"There are people who are dying to help you and all you need to do is reach out."

LETTER TO A TEEN FROM HER FUTURE SELF

Dear Past Self,

There is so much I wish someone had told you.

I wish someone had told you that that feeling you felt, late at night, was an anxiety attack. That you weren't dying. That it wouldn't last more than ten minutes. That you would feel better.

I wish someone had told you that no, it's not normal to hate yourself. That it's not healthy to feel that way about yourself. But also, that it could be worked on.

I wish someone had told you that even though your friends are going through hard things, that doesn't mean their struggles are off-limits to you. It does not make you any less of a friend to express your depressive thoughts even if they feel it too.

I wish someone had told you that talking about it makes so much of a difference. That when the suicidal thoughts and self-harm crept in, telling someone would help. That even though it would be the most terrifying thing you have done, saying those words and hearing the response would make you understand that someone cared.

I wish someone had told you that getting help is the best feeling in the world. That you will feel more in control. That you can let go of the coping mechanisms that have been unhealthy. That when you do have bad days, you will have people to talk to and skills to use. That it truly does help if you can try.

And, I wish someone had told you that you are okay as a person. That you will feel awful sometimes, but that it will get better if you work on it. That you are on a journey, and it's okay if you're still figuring stuff out. That people understand, and you are not alone. That it can get better, as long as you keep talking about it and getting the care you need. And that, even if you feel hopeless inside, there are so many reasons to hope.

—Me from the Future

LETTER TO A TEEN FROM HER FUTURE SELF

To My Younger Self,

I want to start this letter by stating: you will be okay. I promise. You have to continue to believe that there is a reason for everything in life— because there is. I have seen it, time and time again in my 17 years. If things do not go your way, you should reflect on what happened, note down adjustments for next time, and move on. Life lessons are waiting to be learned with every new experience.

As much as you would like to, you will not be able to schedule life down to the very last second. Life doesn't always go the way we hope. You won't be able to mentally prepare yourself for what is to come, either. **Life is complex, it is unexpected, and it is a challenge, but it's the only one you have.**

To help you weather the storm, **a little self care goes a long way.** Be kind to yourself. Surround yourself with positive friends, eat comfort food, and if you need a break, say the word and it's yours. You will find that small pleasures, like blasting music in the car, building sandcastles in your sandbox and coloring with crayola super tip washable markers goes a long way.

You will come to realize that **life is too short to be anything but happy.** Stay true to who you are and remember the person you want to be. Control what you can and let the rest be.

Everything is going to work out in the end, regardless of the path you take to get there.

Take your time. You will get there.

As always,
You are absolutely beautiful.
Never forget. <3.

Love,
Your Future Self

DOS AND DONT'S

In teens' words, what you should and should not do

DOS

"Listen to your body."

"Show yourself the love you get from your family and friends."

"Give yourself time in the mornings or at night that's just for you. Doing my hair and make-up in the morning is sooo important for my mental health."

"Tell yourself something good about yourself before you go to bed."

DONT'S

"Don't try to kill yourself."

"Don't be afraid to reach out."

"Don't let yourself become someone you're not."

"Do not overestimate your own abilities—either in terms of academics or your ability to help your friends through their own mental health crises."

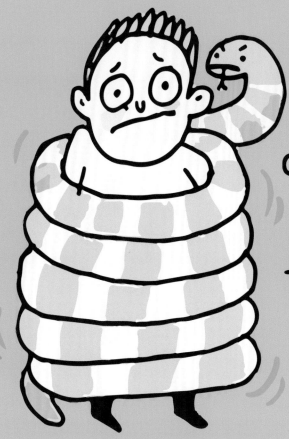

#MENTALILLNESSFEELSLIKE

A BOA
CONSTRICTOR
SLOWLY
SQUEEZING
THE LIFE OUT
OF YOU

@edbites

Gemma CORRELL

PROMOTING TEEN MENTAL HEALTH

What can you do to promote teen mental health?

With their firsthand experience, teens can do a lot to promote teen mental health. We asked teens what they thought.

"Talk about it! Mental health is just as important as physical health. Just because you can't see it, doesn't mean it doesn't exist."

Acknowledging the issue is always the first step to fixing it. Teens also shared some other insights.

"Help those in need, but do it out of understanding...and not out of pity."

Teens also agreed on the importance of being honest and reaching out to others to talk about their issues.

"Be honest about when I'm not okay, rather than just saying 'I'm good' all the time. This will help reduce the stigma that is deterring people from getting the help they need and deserve."

Teens agree—even baby steps towards promoting teen mental health can make a huge impact.

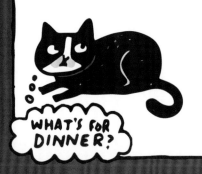

RESOURCES

RESOURCES AND CRISIS NUMBERS

Resource Name	Contact Information
American Foundation for Suicide Prevention (AFSP)	afsp.org
CHC Clinical Services	chconline.org/teens 650.688.3625 caremanager@chconline.org
Crisis Text Line	Text HELLO to 741741
Each Mind Matters - California's Mental Health Movement	eachmindmatters.org
JED Foundation	jedfoundation.org
Lifeline Crisis Chat	suicidepreventionlifeline.org/chat
Mental Health America	mentalhealthamerica.net
National 911 System	911
National Alliance on Mental Illness	nami.org
National Institute of Mental Health	nimh.nih.gov
National Suicide Prevention Lifeline	1.800.273.TALK (8255) suicidepreventionlifeline.org
OnYourMind Teen Chat	onyourmind.net
Strong 365	strong365.org
Suicide Prevention Resource Center	sprc.org
Teenztalk	teenztalk.org
The Trevor Project	1.866.488.7386 thetrevorproject.org

* **24/7 resources for mental health emergencies.** If you or someone you know is in crisis, please dial 911, go to the nearest emergency room, call 1-800-273-TALK (8255), or text HELLO to Crisis Text Line at 741741. You are not alone.